Tending Your Internal Garden

Dr. Christopher Maloney, N.D.

ISBN: 1507869371

ISBN-13: 978-1507869376

DEDICATION

To all those who came before, fermenting, ageing, and keeping
the diversity of our inner gardens alive.

CONTENTS

ACKNOWLEDGMENTS

I want to acknowledge the extraordinary commitment of the human genome project, which spawned the human microbiome project. I also want to thank the American Gut project, Jeff Leach, and all the tireless medical, biological, and microbiome researchers who are bringing the world of the human microbiome to light.

I also want to thank all those who have seen me as patients, who have taught me so much about what is possible. You are the heroes of your lives and health journeys. Thank you for letting me join you on your journey to health.

WHAT IS YOUR INTERNAL GARDEN?

1

DO YOU HAVE WHAT IT TAKES TO GARDEN?

In modern times, one person may love gardening while another would rather eat fried worms than play with them in the dirt. But unlike soil gardens, few of us have any choice in having an internal garden. We all have one, and whether it is an unruly, terrifying mass of disgusting weeds or an ordered, perfectly manicured set of plants worthy of the palace of Versailles, we need to roll up our sleeves and take charge at some point.

For those without gardening skill, tending to an internal garden can be intimidating. But do not be afraid. All of us have been tending our gardens since we were born. From the first time you projectile vomited onto a hapless parent or blew out your diaper with a massive flow, your garden was actively being cultivated. You were rotating your internal crops rapidly and efficiently despite your parents' hapless screams and protests.

That said, this internal garden is a bit flummoxing for even the most educated PhD in agriculture. We did not even have a true sense of the internal garden, or any means to truly measure it, until about ten years ago. And, unlike a soil garden, the internal garden's growth patterns can shift dramatically within a day. Imagine planting tomatoes and waking the next day under the shade of Baobab trees where your tomatoes used to be. Anyone who has suffered food poisoning knows that the situation down below can change at a moment's notice.

Since the internal garden, dubbed the "microbiome," has been hot news on the health front we will see a range of books dictating which species will be better for you and yours. For the most part try to ignore this overly-generalized advice, just as you would someone telling you how to grow Florida orange trees in Maine. The way to build a successful garden has everything to do with your personal soil and conditions. When we generalize too broadly that one-size-fits-all, we make one-size-fits-no-one.

For those of you with gardening experience, some of this book may be the application of tried-and-true common sense gardening.

For those of you without gardening knowledge, we will be learning the basics as well. Try to retain the equivalent of: "find a sunny spot. Put a seed in the ground. Water well." Beyond that things get more complicated quickly.

The art of gardening is the art of trial-and-error. With your internal garden, the same rules apply. Nothing in this book takes the place of your own experimentation, and your garden will flourish under your watchful eye if you learn to tweak "what should work" to "but this works" as fast as you learn it. So, let's begin!

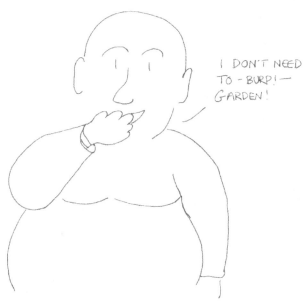

I DON'T NEED TO - BURP! — GARDEN!

2

OF COWS AND MEN

An Historical and Educational Tour

What does it mean when we say something is a "microbiome"? The first part of the word means microscopic, too small to be seen by the naked eye. And a biome is a very large geographic area where plants and animals are similar based on temperatures and weather, like the plains of Africa. So the originators of the word meant to imply something huge when they started using that word. They were talking about something that would change the way we viewed ourselves. The microbiome refers to the immense number of genes contained in our bodies and the microbiota are the creatures who live in us. But for the sake of simplicity, let us call it all the microbiome or, even more simply, our internal garden.

The idea of a microbiome isn't new, but even the idea that bacteria existed and could be the cause of disease hasn't been an easy sell. Back in Greek times, Hippocrates noted that all disease begins in the gut, describing many infectious diseases even though he never saw the bacteria that caused them. In the 1600s, Anthony Leeuwenhoek is credited with the first extensive viewing of what he called "animalcules" swimming in pond water (and in the plaque buildup from his unbrushed teeth). But he didn't make the connection between what was swimming in his plaque and the fact that the plaque itself was the coral-reef-like buildup of their remains. The first well-publicized bacteria-disease connection came in 1847 when Ignaz Simmelweiss tried to stop transmitting bacteria using hand washing. His effort was resisted by prominent doctors of the day. They ridiculed Simmelweiss and eventually had him sent to an insane asylum. It took Louis Pasteur's determination to convince doctors that bacteria did not simply show up spontaneously in patients. Even so, medical handwashing just became standardized worldwide in 1975.

For those of you lathering up with your favorite alcohol antiseptic in response to that history, nothing beats good old soap and water which floods your hands and flushes away much of your load. It would take 97% pure alcohol to sterilize most of the bacteria off your hands (now, that's a recipe for dry, cracked palms). Want to get rid of all the bacteria? It's not possible from any form of washing. They can't even get rid of all the bacteria in NASA clean rooms where they prepare probes to search the universe for signs of life. You can't escape the microbiome.

When we first learn about the benefits of a healthy microbiome, we don't hear that word at all. Probably we learn in grade school about cows. Cows eat grass, and then the bacteria in their four stomachs gradually converts the grass into food for them and yummy milk for us (the Dairy Council funds most of the nutritional education we receive right up through medical school). We all ooh and aah about what an amazing thing cow stomachs are, and usually move on to coloring in a picture of a happy child with lots of milk products.

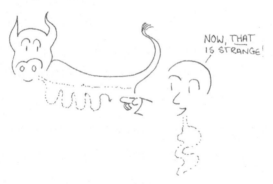

No connection is made between the cow's four stomachs and our own single stomach. A confused or curious third grader might ask why we can't eat grass too, and if the teacher knows she might say we can't digest it because we don't have the enzymes. But the cows don't have the enzymes either. Their bacteria do. The healthy human gut may not digest grass well, but we have bacteria that at least partially digest grass-like fibers.

If we advance in our microbiome education to high school health class, we might learn the different parts of the human digestive tract. The mouth, the esophagus, the stomach, the small intestine, and the large intestine. You might remember that the small intestine, if all its folds were stretched out, would be the size of a tennis court. And, in passing, if your health teacher wanted to gross you out she might mention that there is a lot of bacteria in your poop that helps make vitamins for you. But the focus would likely have been on how much protein is in milk products, and the walls featured athletes with milk mustaches (90% of African and Asian people are lactose intolerant, leading to Lactaid sales and a lot of flatulence as that lactose ferments in the microbiome).

Chances are that's as far as most of us got when it comes to our knowledge of the gut and the microbiome. But say you went on into a health care field. They might have given you anatomy class, where you color in all the parts of the body, including the squiggly small intestine and the larger, looping, large intestine. Maybe you took organic chemistry, where they talked about the complex actions of the body's gut enzymes on dairy products and other food.

If you're in the right medical field, you might even get to look at a cadaver, donated to science, now pink instead of grey from chemical preservatives. Bits and pieces of the human gut would be exposed to your viewing, stuck through with pins and looking like rawhide. The bacteria of the microbiome are ignored as a part of the body, sterilized away by harsh chemicals. It has always been assumed that the bacteria proliferate uncontrollably in the body immediately after death, but they often decrease in both diversity and numbers. Turns out that a microbiome used to living at tropical temperatures doesn't always thrive in a room-temperature corpse.

Say you wanted some hands-on experience with the living microbiome. Even if you took the step of becoming a surgeon, opening up human bodies to reposition and repair, your knowledge of bacteria would be limited to the fact that you don't like them and that you spend your time in fear that the darn gut might rupture and make a mess in what you fool yourself into thinking is a sterile field (remember the NASA clean rooms?). Even though you work with them in your thoughts every day, your knowledge of bacteria would be limited to the risk of infection.

But say that you were really determined to learn about bacteria and the microbiome. You could learn about the known pathological bacteria as a microbiologist. You would learn about bacteria as the enemy, and come up with different ways to kill different species. Most of your knowledge would be limited to a few dozen nasty, lethal creatures capable of causing outbreaks and epidemics.

If you wanted to learn about the microbiome's good bacteria and how to grow a decent internal garden, even fifteen years ago your search would be much harder. If you searched the medical libraries for information, all you would find would be sources like old German monographs discussing the transit time of yogurt through the gut. Physiology texts or nutrition texts might note in passing that beneficial bacteria provide a certain amount of protein and create some B vitamins. Again, our knowledge was limited by the fact that most of the bacteria in the gut are anaerobic, which means they die off in the presence of air. We could check a poop sample for aerobic (air breathing) bacteria, and might know enough that certain species were related to epidemics and other health problems. But these were only the few that survived in the poop when exposed to air. Everything else, almost all of it, was completely unknown. Nobody really thought about the gut unless it acted up.

All that changed when we started being able to analyze the DNA of the unexplored and unculturable areas of the gut. Computer technology advanced enough to allow the processing and matching of massive amounts of raw data, Without that ability there wasn't any way to analyze the genetics of the dead gut bacteria effectively. So when we talk about microbiome research, we are talking about a field that is only about ten years old. Prior to that, research was limited to the outside edges, the top of the gut and the bottom. We could read the cover of the microbiome book, but not the book itself.

Now we're just starting to get an idea of what lies inside us, and it is far more important and complex than anyone realized. It's not a stretch to say that the inner garden of the microbiome defines illness and disease. The uniqueness of our individual microbiomes is assured as "a single host gene can have a tremendous effect on the diversity and population" of the microbiome. Even as the microbiome defines us, we define it.

3

WONDERLAND

WE DO NOT TRAVEL THROUGH LIFE ALONE.

You are a wonderland. Not metaphorically, literally a wonderland. Yes, I'm speaking about you, dear reader. If I could poke my finger out of this book I would prod you gently in the belly and smile like Willy Wonka throwing open his Chocolate Factory doors. Within you there thrives an ecosystem that stretches back to the dawn of time. Again, not figuratively, literally. Bacteria once thought to have died off hundreds of thousands of years ago have been found in the human gut. Strange bacteria that are only found on thermal vents deep in the ocean have been found inside the body. If Jurassic Park had been filmed in your belly, they wouldn't have had to fake the dinosaurs.

We are not alone, and those who travel with us all our days outnumber our cells by at least ten to one. Our DNA, a paltry twenty-three thousand genes, is dwarfed by the genetic material of those we carry with us - ten million genes strong. If we're comparing in technological terms, our genetic code is a calculator and our internal garden is a supercomputer.

The strangest aspect of all this is that we are just "discovering" it for the first time. Advances in DNA testing have allowed researchers to begin to track the microbiome or ecosystem within. But we are just brushing the surface, and researchers believe that over half of what they find is genetic "dark matter" that we cannot identify. We are a mystery.

You are a product of your environment, but that environment extends back to everything you've ever come into contact with or eaten. Once you've come to a stable state, you have your own unique ecosystem. No two internal gardens, like no two snowflakes, are ever the same.

As we travel through the amazing world that is you, we will begin to point out the different groups of your inner dwellers. It may feel as we go that we have labeled you and defined what you are inside. Nothing could be further from the truth. When I say something like: "most of us are mostly firmicutes (pronounced firm-e-cuties)" I have not said anything more specific than: "most of the things that fly are birds." Firmicutes include everything from familiar lactobacillus acidophilus (found in most yogurts) to life-threatening clostridium difficile (an antibiotic-resistant bacteria). Within your body are 16,000 different species, 70% of which are specific to you alone. This is true even of identical twins, even if they live in the same house and are licked by the same dog. You are unique.

4

RAINFOREST

If you understand that your own body contains an incredibly varied and complex ecosystem that is 70% unique to you alone, then you might get a sense of the magnitude of what we're dealing with and why so many scientists are excited about what we're finding.

Imagine walking along what you thought was a well-worn path to your house, looking left, and seeing the entire Amazon rainforest basin stretched out before you, somehow sandwiched between the baseball field and Mr. Johnson's old RV. That's what is going on in biomedical circles right now. They thought they knew everything they needed to know about the gut, and it turns out they missed the entire Amazon rainforest. All the things true of a rainforest apply: thousands of uncatalogued species, completely uncatalogued organisms, and the possibility of finding cures for currently incurable diseases.

Have a look down at your own belly. It's all in there. And you just thought you were ordinary. It turns out that you are an irreplaceable international treasure. We don't know what's inside you, and you may carry a species that is not replicated anywhere else on earth. Somewhere inside you, perched just south of your sphincter of Oddi, could be a bacterial colony that contains the world's best antibiotic, the secret to reversing diabetes, or a harmless method for cleaning oil spills. We don't know. Currently research firms are trying to patent compounds identical to those common in the human gut as new antibiotics.

As we begin to explore, some of these species inside you may sound familiar. We have lactobacillus, a bacteria you may have seen listed as an ingredient in any yogurt. Lacto- means milk-eating and bacillus=bacteria. These bacteria love milk and turn it into yogurt. But they also populate the human gut, either passing through as part of your meal or setting up along the many ridges that make up your intestines. yogurt comes in, populations rise. So far, it doesn't sound that complicated.

But just because we know the family name, lactobacillus, doesn't mean that we know that much about the bacteria in your gut. Different members of the same family, lactobacillus acidophilus or lactobacillus casei, can act very differently in the gut and can have completely different interactions with the bacteria already living there.

Beyond lactobacillus, most of these larger bacterial groups, firmicutes (the group that includes both lactobacillus and clostridium), bacteriodetes (includes our first bacteria, bifida species) and the rest, should sound like a lot of Latin. Is it important to know all the group names? Not really. Because at this point we have no real idea if they are important. Simply because we know the group name and the family name doesn't mean that we know what a particular species is doing in your gut. You might remember that the name for an Australian crocodile is Crocodylus johnstoni, but what you really want to know is how aggressive it is and how fast it can run. Right now we have no idea if the name of the bacteria means anything in terms of what it actually does in our guts. Even if we knew that about a particular gut species, we have no idea how it is interacting with other species.

As the media, diet gurus, and fitness experts get a little more familiar with gut bacteria, we will see a lot of claims and conjectures without a lot of evidence. Think of it like nutrition at the turn of the 20th century, when there was really still cocaine in Coke and people sold all sorts of things based on the little they knew about what was going on in the body. Currently, some researchers are making a lot of noise about the fact that people who are obese have more firmicutes than bacteriodetes. But those who promote a meat-based diet (which seems to promote more firmicutes) are quick to point out that we don't know which species of firmicutes are more active. And the species really matters, because a vegetarian diet gives you more growth of the clostridium family, not the bad, antibiotic-resistant kind, but another species that might help prevent the bad kind from getting a foothold.

One thing to remember in all this is the 70% number in your personal rainforest. What makes up the majority of your personal biome is yours alone. This "uni-biome" (or unique biome) is yours, and anyone claiming to have the answers for your system has never walked a mile in your...you get the picture. So any advice about the nature of what should be happening in your system is likely to not address your terrain adequately. The comparison would be trying to use a greenhouse guide to grow plants in the Maine woods. It might work, but it might not go anywhere because the conditions are fundamentally different.

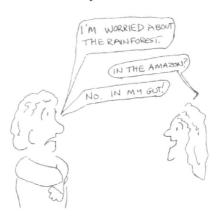

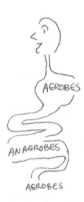

5

A BIRD'S EYE VIEW

Even though we know very little, we know enough to talk about some of the larger groups in your microbiome garden. These are important because they will clarify what might and might not work when tending your garden. So let's focus on the larger groups with an eye to thinking about improving the garden.

Let's start with the two classes of bacteria on and in your body. We have aerobes (oxygen breathers) and anaerobes (for whom oxygen is deadly). Think of these as the sun lovers and the shade plants of the internal garden. Naturally, the aerobes make up most of the garden where air travels: your skin, your nose, mouth, down into your stomach and the beginning of your small intestine. They also make up a good quantity of your bacteria at the other end, where you are again open to the air That's the anus, rectum, and the lower part of the large intestine. The part in the middle is full, typically, of more anaerobes who don't need the oxygen and flourish where there isn't any. The anaerobic territory covers most of the small intestine and some of the large intestine.

Most of what we know about the garden is confined to the oxygen-loving aerobes. They are the ones that we could see, that we could grow in petri dishes and in culture to check for illness. Aerobes are bacteria that we're used to seeing and dealing with. They make up the minority of the total, because most of the gut isn't open to the air. The anaerobes are more numerous and far more mysterious. We've always known they were there, but until we had the ability to categorize them we greatly underestimated their diversity, complexity and sheer numbers.

Our aerobic and anaerobic classes can be broken down into different families: firmicutes, bacteriodetes, etc. (These are actually phylum, but we're ignoring strict naming to help anyone without a PhD in biology get the general idea.) These families are only one way to classify bacteria, and microbiologists prefer to define bacteria based on whether or not they stain well with gram stain. Gram positive bacteria stain purple with Gram's violet dye, while Gram negative bacteria stain pink with a second dye. For the purposes of something like the internal garden whether a bacteria stains well matters a lot less than whether it likes open air. But just be aware that the term gram-negative means a bacteria doesn't stain well because it's a little more complicated. Those wanting more of a background in microbiology can look at classic texts, which give a great deal of information that deals with individual bacteria and much less with their group interactions.

Some of the more familiar families of air breathing aerobic bacteria will be streptococcus (remember strep throat?), staphylococci (skin infections), and enterococci (that can cause food poisoning). As aerobes these species are unlikely to be major players in the gut rainforest because there isn't enough air down there. They are also gram-positive species, which means they stain well and have a thinner wall that may make them easier to kill with antibiotics. One of the current issues in medicine is that both staphylococci (skin) and enterococci (gut) are trading genetic information and making themselves antibiotic resistant. Streptococcus hasn't done as well at developing resistance, which is why a strep infection will likely still respond to amoxicillin, one of the oldest antibiotics.

Deep in the gut are the anaerobes, which previously only included a few families. Clostridium is here, which may not sound familiar until we mention a couple of notorious family members; Clostridium tetani (cause of Tetanus) and Clostridium botulinum (Botulism, which used to be deadly and is now a wrinkle treatment). We're all fortunate that these don't like air and are limited to areas where they aren't exposed. But there are numerous species of this family and lesser known families like Actinomyces and Bacteroides.

Then there are the families that like air, but can stand it when there isn't much around. These are called "aerobic facultative anaerobes." Happier in the air, but capable of living without it if they need to. A lot of our familiar families are here: e. coli, salmonella, krebsiella, shigella, and good old lactobacillus. Different members of this group prosper under different conditions, so it is likely that that battle for the inner rainforest hinges in part on the amount of air and who is exposed to it.

Just when your head was spinning about all the different players, let's be clear that we haven't covered the smaller bacteria, the fungi, or the viruses that make up the rainforest floor. We don't know how these interplay with the larger bacteria and species. Think of what we've covered this far as pointing out where the trees change over to a different dominant species. Up there on the skin and mouth mountains we have a bunch of air breathers. Then as we get down into the throat foothills we get a transition to more of our switch-hitters that can do either air or no air. As we come into the valley of the gut, we switch again to mostly non-air breathers. Below that bacterial canopy we have a whole new world of fungal shrubs and stunted proteobacteria bushes. Under them we have the ground cover of unknown viruses. That's the birds-eye view so far.

6

IS IT REALLY A RAINFOREST?

When we think about a rainforest, we think about a range of plant and animal species. But what we are taught about bacteria is that they are all in it for themselves. How could they not be? They are simple, one-celled organisms that have only rudimentary awareness. Sure, they might be attracted to a food source, but only for themselves. The only way they work together is by mobbing the food source and overwhelming it by sheer numbers. Each of them is only interested in itself. Our image of them is like little zombies. They are all going after us all the time, and we should just kill them off for their own good. That image is wrong.

We've known about biofilms for a while. These darn "zombie" bacteria sometimes secrete a film around themselves to protect them from antibiotics and to help them stick to the gut wall. Just a variation on self-interest and self-protection. But an analysis of biofilms shows a distinct separation of labor. Different bacteria maintain the wall, others get food, others reproduce. We don't just have one species contained within a biofilm, we can have several. They seem to be working together.

Other researchers deny that the biofilms are anything other than an artifact. They point to biofilms where different species are trying to destroy each other. It's still a war down there, with a winner-takes-all-the-food-and-space mentality.

But a study of e. coli brings the "in it for me alone" idea to an end. Faced with ever-increasing amounts of antibiotic, only rare mutant e.coli are resistant. If they were in it for themselves, they would busy themselves in eating everything in sight and forget the rest. Darwinian survival of the species. But instead of focusing on themselves like we would expect them to, the mutants secrete indole, which promotes growth and healing for the other e.coli around them. They do this instead of growing themselves, and making indole takes up much of their energy. Lest we poo-poo this behavior as a byproduct of their mutated state, indole production has nothing to do with their antibiotic resistance.

Why would a resistant e.coli produce healing growth factor for surrounding e.coli? It would do so only if it was aware of its surroundings, and cared enough about those surroundings to change its normal behavior. The surrounding e.coli that the mutants were helping were all relatives, and the researchers called the behavior "kinship" awareness.

To recap, our image of bacteria as wandering, brainless bags of self-interest doesn't match the complexity of what we're seeing on the rainforest floor. We have communities of different species segregating activities in a tribal manner, sometimes getting along and sometimes at war with each other. But within a single species we have displays of altruistic behavior that show a level of awareness and decision-making previously considered inconceivable for a single-celled organism. A rainforest indeed.

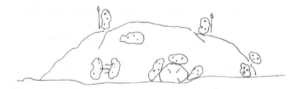

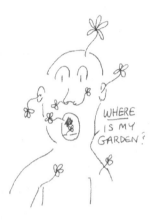

7

WHERE IS MY GARDEN?

Up to this point, I've given the false impression that your garden is contained in the gut. Most of us would also include the skin in the garden, as we are all familiar with hand-washing to keep the bacteria at bay. So we'd place the garden in the belly and on the skin at first glance.

It may come as no surprise to include the nose and lungs in that garden mix. The nose is absolutely filthy with bugs and fungus, containing a honeycomb of smaller bones that warm the air coming in but also provide a trellis for any bacteria wishing to take up residence. While most of us know that someone can get bacterial infections in the lungs (known as pneumonia) few of us realize that there is a constant population of bacteria in the lungs at all times, regardless of our health state.

So the gut, the skin, the lungs, and the nose. That's it, right? Haven't we all been trained think of bacteria as being separate from ourselves? If you get a cut, you put on an antibiotic. You don't want the sterile blood to become infected by bacteria. But what if there were already bacteria in there? Over a nine year period both diabetes and healthy controls had bacteria in their blood, mostly from the family of proteobacteria. These weren't sick people, they didn't have infections, but they did have bacteria living in their blood.

There are areas of the body more important than the blood. We have a set of cells that make up a blood-brain barrier, a final defense for our central nervous system. But this defense is weaker in bacteria-free mice, meaning that having bacteria somehow strengthens those defenses. The bugs in your gut can also directly impact your mood by using your nerves, signaling distress or rest through your own nervous system.

Even if the brain is compromised, one would assume there is one area that is kept completely safe: The placenta of a growing baby should keep all bacteria away. Except that it doesn't. Previous studies tied bacterial growth to birthing difficulties, but researchers checking the placenta for bacteria found that 27% of mothers had bacterial growth there without any effect on the birth process.

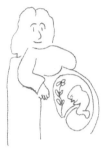

So perhaps the entire body has bacteria involved somewhere, but when something like an artificial hip is transplanted into the body, that is at least sterile, right? No, unfortunately hip transplants can be covered with the oddest bacteria, some of which are usually only found near deep sea thermal vents.

Before we all go out to yell at our surgeons for poor hygiene, even in NASA "clean rooms" where they prepare robotic spacecraft to go out in search of signs of life in the universe you can still find bacterial species. These have been exposed to radiation, burned with acid, frozen, smothered in salt, and torched. Yet a wide variety continue to exist. Can we really expect any area of our bodies to be more sterile?

Once we've concluded pretty much every area of our body is affected by bacteria, (and none of it can be sterilized completely clean) shouldn't that be the end of the garden? No, it's just the beginning. Let's look at other gardens that exist within and alongside the microbiome garden. These are virtually unknown, but promise to change the way we view ourselves even farther.

8

THE MYCOBIOME

What's a mycobiome? The study of funguses in the human body. Not just as disease-causing nasty invaders, but also as possible aids in the our internal garden. In some studies of fungi, they worsen diseases of the gut. But allergic noses do better with many different types around to prevent the allergen from taking over. And other studies say that fungi being around doesn't make any difference. You might just have a fungal growth that isn't causing any problems.

The lion's share of what we know about our internal gardens is based on bacteria. They make up the research. A search for "microbiome" on bacteria turns up over ten thousand articles, a search on "mycobiome" on fungi in the body comes back with less than fifty.

The problem is that we aren't thinking about fungi as being generally helpful, so the research isn't be cataloged properly. My favorite yeast, S. boulardii, has almost five hundred studies that don't appear if you are looking for mycobiome information. Yeast is technically a one-celled fungi, vaguely related to the mushroom. But because in medicine they don't think of yeasts as fungi, studies on yeast aren't included as mycobiome research. They also don't think of cheeses as fungi. So when medical researchers investigate the "French Paradox" (high fat diet/low cholesterol) and think that cheese intake may have something to do with it, that also doesn't count toward mycobiome research.

The human body certainly contains fungi, and many different species. The question is whether these are of no importance, a nuisance, or beneficial. Specifically, given our poor twenty-three thousand genes, can we utilize our internal fungi as endophytes (a mutually beneficial relationship) to provide us with a greater range and function? If a plant can increase its root web by seventy times using endophytes, what about the human body? We certainly consume endophytes within plant matter, as most known plants have some endophiles. If we didn't utilize these supportive fungi, or if our bacteria didn't utilize those fungi for us, that would be a very inefficient system.

Unfortunately, fungi are still seen as either the causes of disease or simply present. When a study noted that a species of pneumonia-causing fungus existed in a healthy individuals, they simply mentioned it to help others determine better what species was causing the pneumonia rather than asking if that fungus could have been doing anything helpful. While endophytic compounds have been shown to be effective against cancer, one expert estimated that 95% of endophytes remain undiscovered. But if we acknowledge that all plants contain endophytes, we would expect that many animals would as well. This is an untapped field and one with immense potential beyond the bacterial microbiome.

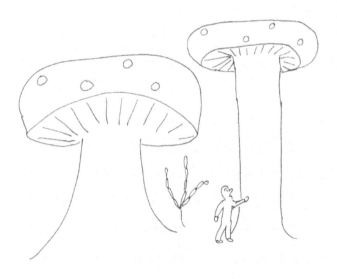

9

THE PATHOBIOME

The last thing anyone wants to think about during surgery is the bacteria on the skin. If we're lucky, we think, we'll avoid an infection. An infection is an overgrowth of a single bacteria, a single species, that we are taught has slipped through the sterile surgical field and occupied our bodies. The only choice in that case is to take lots of antibiotics to kill off that single errant invader.

A surgical infection would more realistically be seen as the overgrowth and domination of a single species within a teeming "pathobiome." Researchers found more than a hundred different species living in supposedly sterile surgical areas, so a sterilized field just means there are less of certain bacteria and more of others. A person wishing to avoid opportunistic, infection-causing bacteria might wish for more diversity in his field rather than more sterility. And it isn't just because those surgeons didn't wash their hands. A study of handwashing in the hospital vs. using an alcohol disinfectant found that neither one was effective at avoiding bacterial colonies on patients. And those just weren't dirty hospitals, as the World Health Organization withdrew two antiseptic cleaners it approved for surgery because they didn't work and now recommends concentrated straight alcohol. It's a futile effort to create a truly sterile field. In comparison, intensive care patients given probiotics had less infection.

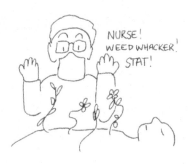

10

THE PALEOMICROBIOME

With the ability to sequence the microbiome, a new field called "paleomicrobiology" has sprung up. By analyzing fossilized poop, these paleomicrobiologists can tell us that the microbiome from over a thousand years ago bears more similarities to hunter-gatherer societies than our own modern guts.

Those engaging in the diet wars (vegan vs. paleo, etc.) will likely try to use any results to support their points of view. What are we to make of the fact that we've been eating corn for over a thousand years? Depending on your diet beliefs it means either that 1000 years ago human beings were already on the decline, or they had figured out that grains are good (as long as they're organic and grown by farmers who get paid well). In this field every discovery will be highly political and likely publicized beyond what is reasonable (the corn study had two fossilized participants).

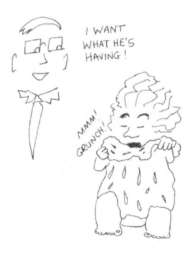

11

THE PARASITOME?

While most of us would gladly down a few probiotics, few of us would take parasites. But an analysis of chimpanzees found their guts teeming with parasites that performed a variety of internal functions. Have a look at all their parasites: Troglodytella abrassarti, Troglocorys cava, Blastocystis spp., Entamoeba spp., Iodamoeba butschlii, Giardia intestinalis, Chilomastix mesnili, Bertiella sp., Probstmayria gombensis, unidentified strongylids,

Strongyloides stercoralis, Strongyloides fuelleborni, and Trichuris sp.

Without our own endemic parasites, what is missing from a civilized man's diet? Should we look for hookworm in a bottle? Add it to our morning vitamins and supplements?

When we think of something like Giardia lamblia we think of infection (or we think, huh? because we have blissfully never encountered this particular parasite in stream water). But despite the standard assumption of bloody diarrhea and Flagyl treatment, it is perfectly possible to simply be a carrier of Giardia lamblia without any symptoms.

Something a little less common in humans, Strongyloides stercoralis (round worm or thread worm), may be in the human gut for a lifetime without presenting symptoms. Even if it is suspected, it may take <u>seven</u> different stool analyses to catch an infection. While officially someone would need to walk barefoot on poop-infected ground to get round worm, a hospital water survey found it in the drinking water (it wasn't the hospital's fault because the lake water that the entire town was using was infected). Before we all go avoiding that one town, an estimate puts poop contamination in the water of one in three people (while rates are higher in some parts of the world, you can get a contaminated glass almost anywhere). A person might die, donate his or her organs, and then the recipient can come down with a Strongyloides round worm infection because the immune suppressing drugs let the parasites grow like crazy. But in some sick patients, having Strongyloides infections might even be beneficial. Infected Ugandan HIV patients with a parasitic infection got worse slower, not faster. Those with ongoing parasitic infection had lower HIV virus counts. Another study of Australian aborigines found that those infected with Stongyloides were 61% less likely to have diabetes. But these studies are few and far between, because we overwhelmingly treat parasites as if they were always a bad situation for the internal garden. Regardless of their possible worth, I doubt we'll see "probiotic" parasites anytime soon.

12

THE VIROME?

When they analyzed human guts, the whole place was teeming with viruses. Disturbingly, most of these viruses did not match any known virus. So our guts are teeming with viruses that haven't even been named yet.

Are they important? They can kill a baby. Women who miscarry often have an overgrowth of a bacteria, Trichomonas Vaginalis. While antibiotics can kill off the bacteria, killing the bacteria does not improve the ability of infected women to have babies. Researchers identified a virus that lives inside the Trichomonas bacteria, Trichomonasvirus, that triggers the body to miscarry. The antibiotic used to kill the bacteria inflames the virus, so the women miscarry at the same rate they would if the bacteria was left alone. Since the bacteria infects about two hundred and fifty million women in the world, just that one virus is pretty important and we have hundreds. Another circumstance where a different model of garden tending is critical.

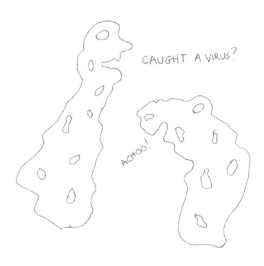

HOW TO TEND YOUR INTERNAL GARDEN

13

SHOULD I GET MY SOIL TESTED?

When gardening, one of the basic first steps is to get your soil tested to determine what is missing and what will benefit your plants. Since you are investing serious time into a long growing season, testing your soil before you begin makes sense.

What if the growing season was less than a day, and the entire soil base could shift in that time? Anyone who has endured a Thanksgiving dinner or experienced travelers' diarrhea knows this can be the case. Is it still worthwhile to have your soil checked?

In the case of the human body, we are really discussing your "night soil," your bowel movements, feces - just plain poop. For varying amounts of money, you can have your poop examined by any number of conventional or specialty labs. The Human Microbiome project may not want to look at your poop, but for a donation, the American Gut Project might have a gander (http://americangut.org/). If they don't want it you can get any number of less specific tests done by specialty labs, from the fiber content to how well you're digesting your greens. The costs vary, but you can get a general idea for about a hundred dollars and spend thousands if you really want to dig deeply (ewww!).

If you want a general picture of what your garden looks like, it turns out that the American Gut Project and the Human Microbiome Project overlap nicely. A look at the nicely colored maps on their websites shows that most of us have similar skin, mouth, and poop families. None of them, even in the same individual, overlap that much. So we could really think about our personal gardens as three different gardens: the one in the full sun (skin), the one in partial sun (the mouth) and the one in the shade (gut).

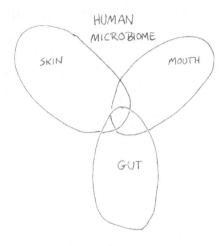

How static these bacteria are in one person, even at the group level, can change dramatically. On his blog, Jeff Leach (who promotes the Paleo diet and the American Gut Project) obsessively tracks his own changes in inner garden families over a move from one location to another and a change in diet. By changing location and having less plants available, he switched from mostly firmicutes (which may make you fat) to mostly bacteriodetes (which may be less likely to make you fat) in the matter of a few months. The only standard garden equivalent would be starting with a Christmas tree farm and ending up with a vineyard after a few months simply by changing your fertilizer. This change compares to Mr. Leach's later trials of himself in Africa, eating and drinking with the natives, culminating in a self-done fecal transplant from a bemused tribesman. (The poor fellow must be wondering about what we like to call civilization these days: "First, they took our land. Then they took our culture. Now they want our poop?"). Both experiments resulted in huge garden shifts, but the less-vegetable change was much less arduous.

So, given the shifting nature of the soil, is it worthwhile to have your soil tested? If you are having difficulty with your soil (chronic diarrhea, irritable bowel, Crohn's, celiac, etc.) then it would be a reasonable idea to have it checked. But if your soil seems reasonably stable and sound, then taking preliminary gardening steps first makes more sense. Test the soil later on if you run into difficulty, or do it now if you really believe you don't fall within the standard mapping and need to be sure.

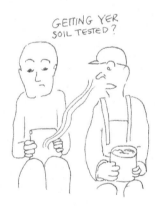

14

BEGINNING A GARDEN

Unless you've just been born (in which case congratulations on being a prodigy already), chances are that you've been internal gardening all of your life. Maybe your garden has been a junkpile full of old pork rinds and milk that spoiled but you held your nose and drank it anyway. Or maybe you swallow lots of capsules and pleasure-free food on a given day as some kind of personal, fear-based "health insurance policy." In either case, you're gardening.

We need to garden consciously. The conscious part is a change. No one is asking for you to garden differently, just to take note of the effect your behavior has on your garden. Take note of a post-binge hangover and vomiting episode, and you might consider cutting back on the jello-shots next weekend (better write yourself a note now). Those three full lemon meringue pies may look great going in, but the next fourteen hours on the throne might indicate that the garden isn't pleased by that fertilizer. Unlike the visible garden out behind the house, the inner garden has to make its displeasure known in more physical ways. Wilting and looking pale won't work, but grumbling and flooding the system with liquid might get your attention.

The first step to gardening is to plan a menu. Yes, there are literally hundreds of thousands of different enriching additives that you can put into your garden, with a few hundred new ones coming out every month. But this year you will average two pounds of sugar intake per day, so unless you're buying your supplements and vitamins by the shovelful, chances are very high that what you eat will have the most effect on your garden. Some estimates put the overall consumption of food at somewhere over a ton a year, with 10-20% of that ending up in landfills because we don't have a good handle on how hungry we are.

Most of us have a relatively stable menu that we consume. Yes, there are holidays and visits with parents, but for the most part your diet is pretty stable. Back when there were just a few food groups (dairy, meat, grain, fruit, and vegetable) only one in three people in the U.S. consumed something from all the food groups on a given day. Less than 3% consumed the recommended amounts, and that was when the amounts were much easier to remember. When we switched from the Food Pyramid to My Plate things didn't get much better.

American diets are out of balance with dietary recommendations
In 2012, Americans consumed more than the recommended share of meat and grains in their diets but less than the recommended share of fruit, dairy, and vegetables

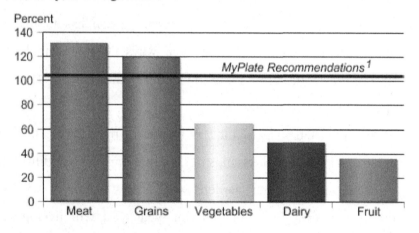

Note: Rice and durum flour data were discontinued and thus are not included in the grains group. Food availability data serve as proxies for food consumption.

[1] Data based on a 2,000-calorie diet.

Source: Calculated by ERS/USDA based on data from various sources (see Loss-Adjusted Food Availability Documentation). Data as of February 2014.

But before you go out and get a Myplate calculator, book, or app for changing your diet realize all those recommendations are likely to change dramatically in the next few years. And remember the "70% rule" because none of the PhDs in D.C. have any idea of what is happening in your personal garden. It doesn't help to dramatically try and change your garden based on someone else's incomplete view of what your garden should look like based on data from years ago which didn't even know the microbiome existed.

If you don't have the time to make a list of what you eat, be happy that your grocery store has done it for you. Ask for your grocery receipts, cringe at the rising cost of food, and take a gander at what you've purchased as fertilizer for this week. A quick look at my own bill gives me some confusion (how many foods are in hummus?) Assigning the number five for every "mixed" food (prepared food, mixed vegetables, etc.) and the number one to every single food (cucumbers, maple syrup, raisins), chances are the total number of foods on your grocery receipt is less than a hundred for the week. That's the extent of your fertilizer diversity.

What else is out there for choices? When researchers charted the diets of people in the U.S. from 1971-75, they tracked 3,462 different individual foods. In the second study in 1991, they tracked 7,096 individual foods.

How does your grocery store list add up? Chances are that week-to-week, you are eating the same foods over and over and over. If you're happy with where your garden is, then you've likely already found a recipe for the right fertilizer. If you're not happy with how your garden is doing, then there's a lot of room to change the fertilizer you use before you shift to additives for your cure. Your gardening might simply begin by turning down an unexplored aisle in the grocery store, holding your breath, and trying something new.

15

HOW DO I KNOW
HOW MY GARDEN IS DOING?

Since our inner garden is inside us, it's a little harder to see. You may be wondering how you know you need more watering if you can't see the leaves wilting. There are those of you that already have diagnoses like Irritable Bowel or Crohns. You know that your garden isn't terribly happy. But unless you have had serious issues it can be a little harder to know where you stand.

When you garden, you have to get your hands dirty. Your internal garden is no exception, except that you may not have to use your hands. You will have to use your eyes, ears, and nose. (If you want a soil sample, you'll be using your hands as well.)

If your neighbor's garden was surrounded by a high wall, but it reeked in there and the fertilizer bin outside the fence was full of rotting vegetables covered in mold and swarming with every kind of pest, you wouldn't need to see inside to know things weren't going well. We have a similar situation in our bodies. Every day you get a chance to see what ends up in the fertilizer bin.

Yes, we're talking about your poop. You may not want to be eating during this next part.

How is your poop these days? If you are one of those people who wipe and run away holding your breath, chances are that you have an issue that you're not dealing with. If you clear the room, the hallway, and the office floor with the potency of your personal explosions, chances are that some well-meaning colleague has gifted you this book and highlighted this sentence. We need to talk.

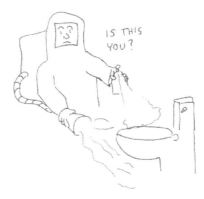

No poop smells that great, but you should be able to stand your own, and the odor should be gone within a minute or two of flushing with the fan on. Depending on your diet, your gas should be either less smelly and more plentiful (typically lots of vegetables) or more smelly but less often (typically more meat, less fiber). If your smell is reasonable it's time to see if you have good-looking poop.

What is a good-looking poop? If you've ever seen a dog pooping or a cow pooping, we're aiming for something in the middle. A dog has a short pipe, and a healthy dog has massaged the poop to the point where it has outlines of the bowel muscles imprinted on it. That's a little too dramatic and dry for us humans. At its worst on the dry end, the poop is so concentrated it comes out in pellets like a rabbit. This is not ideal and your bowel is not likely to be very happy with you.

Compare a dog's offering to a cow's dung. Having done my time in a cow barn, commercial cows all tend toward diarrhea (whether that's natural for cows is another thing). Normally the grain and hay is ejected in gouts of liquid that need to be dealt with using a shovel rather than a rake. If your poop is consistently more like a soup than a solid, then we've got to talk.

What is the ideal poop? If you believe Dr. Oz, there is a poop scale and a consistency that is ideal. He's taken the time to provide a short video on the subject (Just look up Dr. Oz and healthy bowel). Dr. Oz is really just dramatizing the Bristol stool scale, which was created by feeding volunteers either a laxative or a constipating agent and checking it against the shape of the poop. Turns out the shape gives you some idea of how fast things are going through you and whether your garden is irritated (too fast) or too dry (slow). Our ideal is formed and solid, but not imprinted. Think of something like a brown banana (now you'll never eat bananas again).

But what is missing from Dr. Oz's discussion and the Bristol scale is how often a poop should happen. If you believe popular media, anything from three times a day to three times a week is normal. Graphing the bowel patterns of supposedly healthy children and adolescents gives anywhere from 2.4 hours to 86 hours for food to travel through the gut. But adults with disabilities show a much slower bowel movement time, and both constipated and control patients have much shorter bowel movement times after being cleaned out. So if you tend toward the longer end of the spectrum or the shorter end, it may be worth thinking about trying to shift things a bit. How do you tell what your total transit time is? Eat something like corn (which should occasionally appear untouched at the other end unless you chew very well) or beets (which will color everything red as they pass). M.D.s might use a radioactive dye, but you can swallow a charcoal tablet (making everything black) for a home check. The bottom line is that if your stool is formed correctly, it's likely moving through at the unique speed that's right for you.

O.K., you've got your grocery list, you've looked in the bowl, and you've got some sense of how often you go. Where do you start changing your garden? Is it the same as when you go to the greenhouse and buy seeds? Or should you go out and get some wild plants, maybe from the side of the road, to help get things started?

16

TAKING STOCK OF THE CURRENT CROP

Where do you start changing your garden?

Maybe you shouldn't. If things are going well, you have a healthy poop, and you don't have any complaints, then leave yourself alone.

Let me say that again, backed by every patient I've ever seen with horrendous bowel complaints. If it isn't broken, don't fix it. We are living in the stone ages of internal gardening, and we do not understand the complexities of what we're dealing with. So be grateful, thank the universe for not gifting you with this particular problem, and go about dealing with other issues.

Is it the same as when you go to the greenhouse and buy seeds?

Please, no. Without understanding your soil, the current crop, and how you react to new species, buying random seeds and throwing them down into your garden might do nothing, might help, or might lead to explosive consequences.

Let me share a personal story that may help convince you not to go out shopping for the exotic probiotic flavor-of-the-month (Ooh, look honey! They have Akkermansia on sale!).

Back in the pre-stone ages of internal gardening, my instructor told the class that everyone -absolutely everyone- could benefit from this particular high-potency probiotic mixture. Unlike standard probiotic "seed" blends, this particular mixture came in a "sachet" rather than a capsule. The easiest equivalent would be to take an entire bottle of probiotic capsules and pull them apart to leave the powder in a small pile. That pile would be one sachet.

A young and enthusiastic student with no bowel complaints (yours truly) decided that everyone benefitted from probiotics. Why shouldn't I reap the health benefits of this wonderful stuff? It didn't matter that I had no bowel complaints. Probiotics helped with a laundry list of possible complaints and I tend toward the "fear-based, health insurance" model of supplementation. I took a sachet and waited eagerly for the results, which were loud, smelly, and unpleasant all around. It felt like I'd swallowed a gremlin, or at least a grumpy butt gnome (patent pending).

The next time I saw my wise professor, I told him my results. A truly wise student might have taken the results as evidence that not everything my professor said was true. But I was convinced that my professor knew everything (just like many people think their doctors know everything). My professor heard my results and waved them away. "You just didn't do enough." Remember, I had already taken the equivalent of a bottle of probiotics. But I felt ashamed that I hadn't realized my seemingly obvious error. My professor and I both fell into the medical trap of "more is better." In hindsight, I know that in medicine more is almost never better.

That weekend, which went down in my personal history as "the weekend of the six sachets" serves warning to us all about the myth of more is better. I began, as my professor instructed, by taking two sachets of probiotics. I wouldn't be caught unprepared this time, and had four more as backup just in case double the dose was not sufficient. As my abdominal distress mounted, I stubbornly continued to pour sachet after sachet into my fermenting, disturbed belly. Even writhing in flatulent agony, I remember pouring in that final sachet. Somehow I was going to improve my gut, despite this "healing crisis." In hindsight, I recognize that any true healing crisis arises from the body (taking care of a virus, or food poisoning, for examples) and that anyone should discontinue anything that makes them feel this bad. The "healing crisis" is too often a misnamed "I gave you too much and now you have side effects" and I'd like to see it fade from common usage.

On Monday, I confronted my professor with details about my weekend. He looked at me and said: "I don't believe you." That was it. That is how very smart, very well-trained people with medical degrees deal with something that completely goes against what they believe. They simply don't believe it. I've seen it again and again, in every field. Patients need to understand this medical blind spot that can keep them from getting well.

So please, please do not try to "improve" a happy stomach, and if you do add in new seed do it slowly and with the caution you apply to a first meeting with a large and possibly surly dog.

Should you go out and get some wild plants, maybe from the side of the road, to help get things started?

If things are going well, leave the current crop alone. But wild plants will show up from time to time. Usually your body will jettison the invader with diarrhea, but sometimes they set up shop and now you've got an issue that you need to resolve. Then you've got a reason to try to change things around. Happy garden, leave it alone. Unhappy garden, make changes.

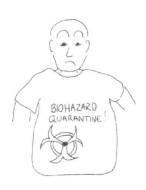

17

STARTING WITH ANTIOBIOTICS:
USING A FLAMETHROWER?

It can be enticing to try and "clear the area" and start your garden with antibiotics. After all, if you want to lay down a new garden shouldn't you clear the land first?

The difficulty here is that we're talking about a rainforest, not a lawn. And unlike our Amazon basin that can't keep up with our bulldozers, our internal gardens can grow as fast as we cut. So let's go through a couple of scenarios on how antibiotics might work in your internal garden. The first scenario is from Wired magazine's microbiome article, showing what happens to your internal garden after a round of broad-spectrum antibiotics. Here's the graph:

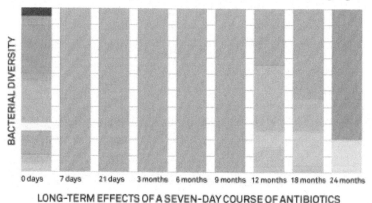

LONG-TERM EFFECTS OF A SEVEN-DAY COURSE OF ANTIBIOTICS

(http://www.wired.com/2011/09/mf_microbiome/)

If you start with an antibiotic, it's like bulldozing down to the bedrock and then waiting for the topsoil to reform. Only if your starting garden is a horrendous, toxic mess (which is more common than you'd think) would you consider starting with antibiotics.

Now, some of the more clever beginning gardeners have the solution to the bulldozed-to- the-bedrock problem. Simply add probiotics, good bacteria, in between the antibiotics. Bulldoze, add grass seed. Bulldoze some more. Instant, perfect garden? Let's look at that as a possibility.

In a study that paired Augmentin, a powerful antibiotic, with a researched probiotic yeast (S. boulardii, which is my current favorite "grass seed"). It was a smart study because about a third of patients develop bad yeast overgrowths after antibiotics. The expectation was that the combination of antibiotic and good yeast would lead to a die off of other bacteria and a bloom of S. boulardii in the gut. That's not what happened.

The good news is that the S. boulardii blocked the expected inflammation of the gut. When antibiotics come through, the cells in charge of setting off autoimmune responses get pretty agitated. That doesn't mean antibiotics cause worsening autoimmune disease, just that they don't help.

But in the combination of antibiotic and S. boulardii, the overall numbers of bacteria in the gut did not change, at least not that they could measure. What changed was the dominant families. On day one of the antibiotic, the members of the Clostridium family dropped, but then increased and continued to increase for the rest of the treatment. Bacteriodes loved the antibiotic and increased until it was stopped. A previously undetected family, Enterobacteriaceae, suddenly came in from out of town and set up shop. When the antibiotic was stopped, that family disappeared into obscurity again. So the S. boulardii, instead of setting up house in the gut, just made the transitions faster. When it was present the families went back to their normal levels sooner than later. So taking S. boulardii with an antibiotic is a good idea to maintain what is in your gut, not to change it.

A few astute readers might notice the outcome of this antibiotic/probiotic maintaining species study is different from the absolute destruction of most bacteria species by an antibiotic shown in the graph on page 59. My response is that individual results may vary widely, and that taking a probiotic with an antibiotic may well help maintain your internal diversity.

So maybe you're convinced to leave the flamethrower in the garage for now. Is it time to go out and buy some seeds? Or maybe we should look at the seeds you have on hand.

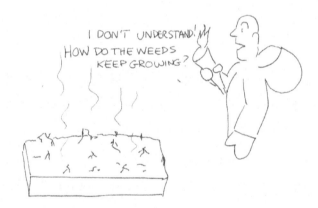

18

PERSONAL WILD SEEDS

Once upon a time we were dirty. Really, really dirty. You may be picturing a cave-dwelling tribe, crouched around the fire, but that's not where the dirty ends.

Despite the Egyptians' use of soap, the Romans never got in the habit. And the Romans were amazingly clean compared to anyone right up through the 17th century, which is thought to be the nastiest time to live in recent history. Europeans were convinced that bathing left someone open to getting more disease (which may not be that crazy) so they left their protective dirt in place their entire lives. The U.S. didn't really catch the clean bug until after the Civil War, when they saw that clean rooms and bedding helped soldiers recover. But even then, families would share a bath, one at a time -in the same water- once a week.

Now, we're all mad for bathing. Everything needs to be cleaner, and we buy antiseptic rinses by the boatload. Washing means less infection, less disease, right? That's the story that we tell ourselves, based on the need for doctors and nurses to clean their hands between sick patients. How does the same advice apply to normal people? It doesn't. Ordinary people who washed their hands more than five times a day were slightly more likely to get a cold than those who washed their hands less often. Would more be better? Increasing washing your hands to more than twenty times a day didn't help at all. So while doctors should wash their hands often, the rest of us may not be helping ourselves with all this extra washing. Even in a situation where everyone would agree absolutely that washing is necessary, right before a surgery, washing the patient's whole body before the surgery did not prevent surgical infections.

So before you go out and purchase seeds, perhaps it's time to look at your hygiene. Particularly your over-abundance of it. If you sterilize your house, your car, and your pets, you might want to start letting them get a little dirty and recognize that you can't make it all go away. Remember that even NASA, who creates clean rooms where they burn, freeze, acid wash, salt, and irradiate the spacecraft they send to other planets to look for bacterial life can't get rid of all the bacteria.

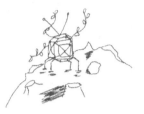

As we say in Maine, "you can't get there from here" meaning you can't get entirely clean. All you're doing on that perfectly bleached countertop is growing the nastiest, toughest bleach-resistant bacteria in your neighborhood. (Oh look, Blanche! I've got botulism spores and a little cluster of tetanus near the toaster!) If they set up shop in your gut, it's just a matter of time before they run into some hospital bacteria (who also thrive in bleach) and start swapping antibiotic resistance. Better to let things slide a little and let a little dust build up in the corners before you spend a lot of money on probiotic grass seed that will look like preschoolers to the Hulk delinquents you've been growing in your three-times-a-day sterilized shower. Let your hair down for a day or two and see what happens first.

Of course, you wouldn't want to collect wild seeds from a waste dump. So cultivate a few good habits. Head to the health food store rather than the we're-all-going-to-die-soon-anyway buffet. Go to the gym rather than the hospital. Expose yourself to the right kind of bacteria, the right kind of situations, and see where that takes you before you start adding in other seeds.

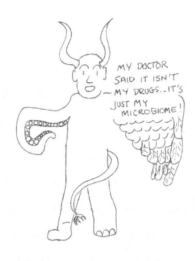

19

MANDATORY FERTILIZER: DRUGS

When we take a prescribed drug, few of us think about the effect on our internal garden. The exception would be when we take antibiotics, and then we might feel bad for our internal garden but think we'll pay it back later with some yogurt. As we pointed out in the flamethrower section, antibiotics don't kill your internal garden, they just change it.

Every other drug does as well. And before we ignore that, the reality is that the internal garden changes the drugs. When given antibiotics, rats absorbed less than half the dose of statin drugs than they would have if they had a fully functioning internal garden. Giving antibiotics to someone on birth control may cause that birth control to fail. Antibiotics can block the bacteria of the internal garden from detoxifying much of the toxins we take in every day.

At the same time, the wrong species in the internal garden may cause a drug to have serious side effects. Flagyl, an antibiotic, is known for its bad side effect picture. But those side effects may be caused by a bacteria, Bacillus thiaminolyticus, that converts Flagyl into a chemical that looks like an essential B vitamin to the body. When the body absorbs this chemical and tries to use it as a B vitamin, all sorts of problems arise.

Few people are in a position to stop their prescriptions. But when side effects occur, talking to your doctor about changing medication is essential. Sometimes patients may think it's all in their heads, but it may just as well be in their guts.

If there's any wiggle room, talk to your doctor about what else you can do to make the medication unnecessary. Chances are that those changes will be good for your gut as well.

20

VOLUNTARY FERTILIZER: SUPPLEMENTS

The same people who might shy away from taking a drug every day may be voluntarily taking a whole range of vitamins, minerals, and miracle-pills-of-the-week. Most believe on some level that what goes in their mouth will end up in their body, not processed by their internal gardens. But that may not be the case.

Taking vitamins does not mean those vitamins are absorbed. In patients with a B vitamin deficiency, taking that vitamin did not resolve their deficiency even after repeating the tests over time.

Once they were given antibiotics, their B vitamin levels returned to normal without supplements. So their deficiency was from an unbalanced garden, not a lack of B vitamins.

Minerals may, in large quantities, act like antibiotics. So a multivitamin with vitamins and minerals may be doing all sorts of indiscriminate feeding and killing as it passes through the system without solving any underlying deficiencies.

Amino acids, the building blocks of protein, feed bacteria directly when taken as supplements. Radiolabelled amino acids end up making radiolabelled bacteria, not radiolabelled big strong muscles. A study on lysine, an amino acid commonly given to help treat herpes outbreaks, found that gut bacteria had over a thousand different new ways of breaking it down. Almost half of those break-down methods had never been seen before in labs. So if you want to feed your bacteria amino acids that's fine, but they may not do much for you. If you really want to get some amino acids past the bacteria, you'd better take enough that you saturate their appetites and bit gets through.

There are so many herbs, and many of them act as antibiotics in the gut. That doesn't mean they kill off all the bacteria, only that they change it dramatically. Much of what we thought was happening from taking herbs may be happening in the gut, not the rest of the body. A few herbs, like green tea, may support more bacterial growth of good bacteria.

Patients taking a vitamin, mineral, herb, or any supplement will be unlikely to be dissuaded by any thought of their inner gardens.

They are looking for a body effect for themselves, defined without the bacteria in mind. And clearly in large enough quantities these do get through the wall of the gut and have an effect. But if a dosage seems too strong or doesn't seem to be doing anything, it is possible that it is simply feeding the gut rather than being absorbed. Not that we don't want to support our friendly bacterial guests. We should just be clear that we are providing a "free lunch" for them first before we reap any direct benefit.

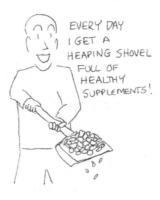

21

VOLUNTARY FERTILIZER: FOOD

Before we step off into the abyss of trying to prescribe a set fertilizer for a planet of "70% unique" human beings who live in vastly different circumstances, let me clarify that we simply don't know what the ideal diet should be - for anyone. And that was before we were thinking about the microbiome at all. If you go to a diet section of a bookstore, you will see variations on the broken idea:

MYTH: **calories in - calories out = weight gain.**

If we expand this to:

CLOSER TO REALITY:

calories in + microbiome breakdown and absorption + hormonal body response + survival set point + starvation accommodation = weight fluctuation and compensation

then we have something more closely approximating the truth, based on what we know in the stone ages of microbiome research. Think of the first equation as the modern equivalent of "fire good!" and the second equation as "fire good unless you're too close or there's a big animal looking for you or there's nothing worth cooking and it's already hot outside." In the meantime, we're traveling around in these high-tech spaceship bodies with no real idea of what we're doing.

Rather than beginning by thinking about adding foods, let's think about taking them away. Not quantity (calories), diversity. Unlike most soil gardens, most human gardeners buy every fertilizer that's on sale and pour it into themselves. If it's even vaguely food-like (think of anything with a shelf-life of two years that hasn't been canned) then we'll eat it. So a beginning food fertilizer plan would be to eliminate many of these excess fertilizers and see if the garden rebels or rejoices.

For those who haven't spent their lives buried in nutritional texts, we're talking about an elimination diet. While the will may be strong, most people respond poorly emotionally to having their favorite foods taken away. For this reason, the diet is repackaged as an "anti-inflammatory diet," justified because most of our common packaged foods are also our most common allergens. A sample anti-inflammatory diet is found in Appendix A at the end of this book. Focusing on what you can eat, rather that what you can't, helps patients comply. Again, there is nothing magical about the foods on the anti-inflammatory diet, which have been selected for what they are not rather than for their own sake. The diet is focused on avoiding common irritants in a western diet, so a Japanese person on a standard Japanese diet might need to alter the diet to avoid all rice, seaweed, and soy products. If you are already on a diet similar to the anti-inflammatory diet, you may need to restrict further. The goal is to fundamentally change your base materials, to really shake things up, and then add back in your common fertilizers to see what's working and what doesn't really matter.

The beauty of the anti-inflammatory diet is that you will not need to wait a growing season to get results. While the traditional anti-inflammatory diet asks that patients hold to the diet for twenty-one days (the minimum time required to truly change a set of mental dietary habits) those using the diet for the purpose of examining the internal garden can begin to add single foods back in within four days (the minimum time required for a shift in gut bacteria).

After four days, adding a food back in requires a fair quantity. A few people will respond to a small amount of the new food, but most require a fair amount throughout the day. Eat a portion at all three meals of the day, in a quantity sufficient to supply a fair amount of the day's calories.

What can you expect if you have a reaction? There are four types of allergic reaction: immediate (now), at absorption (2 hours), when an immune system mounts (a day), and when that immune response needs to be processed (2 days). The immediate response is well-known to allergic individuals with anaphylactic responses who have their tongues begin to swell and require shots of adrenal hormones from epi-pens. One would hope nothing in a person's ordinary diet would cause this response. ("I just love the way the seafood makes my tongue swell?") The second response occurs on absorption and usually happens within two hours of eating. Usually people know what foods "don't agree" with them and avoid those as well. Because the third immune response can take the rest of the day to take effect, many people are not aware that the reason they feel "off" or "really tired" is an allergic food reaction created by the immune response making you feel like you have a touch of the flu.. It may take several days, one day trying the food, another day off the food, to really be certain it is the food that is causing your mood and energy lack. This is equally true of the fourth response, which doesn't show up until the next day when your body feels off or fatigued because it is preoccupied with ridding itself of immune cells combined with the allergen coming out through the kidneys. Many people will miss the connection for years, because the problem-causing food was eaten the day before. They may even show up at the doctor's with ongoing complaints but with no idea what could be causing it.

If you have a response, does that mean you're allergic? No. It's possible that your internal garden is reacting, not your immune system. But something doesn't like that particular fertilizer. So it's best to avoid that food for now, or to eat it only when social pressures compete with your need to have a perfect internal garden (your mother-in-law serves it to you). Because the immune system down-regulates unnecessary responses over time, if you avoid an allergen for six months (the time to turn over most immune cells) it may be possible to have an exposure without symptoms in the future. If you are truly allergic, repeated exposure will likely start up your symptoms again. (You can also be tested for the allergies, but the gold standard test is still elimination and reintroduction).

By focusing on what doesn't bother you, you can find a set of fertilizing meals that you can live on. But in order to thrive, you should expand out your exposures. Eating something new and different once a month is a good practice. If you pay attention to how you feel over the next couple of days afterward, you may find a positive effect, a buoyancy (there is no word for the positive effect that is the opposite of an allergy) from that meal. That's the

73

equivalent of finding a miracle-gro without chemicals for your body. So eat out, eat strangely, and experiment with new fertilizers!

SOMETIMES I THINK MY BRAIN IS AN OLD CALCULATOR BUT MY GUT IS A SUPERCOMPUTER!

22

BUYING SEEDS: THE "MILK" BACTERIA

Before we had the sort of technology we've developed in the last few years that allowed us to check the genetic code of the gut, we only knew about what we could culture at the other end. That limited us to seeing what would survive in the air, which it turns out kills off most of your internal species. That's why, if you look at any books on internal gardening from before the turn of the century (not the 19th century, anything before the year 2000), they wax lyrical about great "crops" of lactobacillus or bifidabacteria. These two still make up almost all probiotics or "internal gardening seeds" on the market today.

But lactobacillus can be either beneficial or possibly inflammatory, depending on the conditions in the gut before applying them. Anyone who has consumed a probiotic drink only to have it ferment embarrassingly for the next few hours will attest that sometimes it isn't better to lay down more seeds.

If you look at the necessary raw materials to grow lactobacillus in the gut, it's not the easiest to grow and maintain. In comparison to something like e. coli, which requires sugar and water, lactobacillus is pretty high maintenance.

When lactobacillus gets together with e.coli, lactobacillus secretes an antibiotic that kills the e.coli so that lactobacillus can harvest it for nutrients. Not quite the gentle milk bacteria we were expecting. That same milk bacteria antibiotic can kill off a range of other bacteria, meaning that adding lactobacillus into a gut may not equate to the increase in bacterial growth we would expect. Lots more milk bacteria, but not much of anything else.

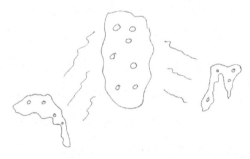

So, we have fewer bacteria, but that's all right. Maybe.

Different species of milk bacteria have different effects on the gut. We're not talking about minor effects. We're talking changes in the genetic structures of the gut lining. Within six hours of taking different lactobacillus species volunteers had "expression of several hundred up to thousands of genes" within their guts. Not only was the individual expression very different, the species of lactobacillus really mattered. Lactobacillus acidophilus (by far the most common supplement) altered insulin, hormones and metabolism. Lactobacillus casei (which is another common yogurt bug) altered genes involved in mitosis, growth, and proliferation. Lactobacillus rhamnosus altered genes involved in wound repair and healing. So depending on the species of milk bug you choose, the results are very different.

All this is hardly surprising to the gardener. Anyone who's shopped for tomato plants knows there are different plants with very different growth cycles even within the commercially available. With a tomato plant you have a single entity that doesn't have to coexist with other plants. Imagine dropping a million tomato plants into wild grass land and expecting a consistent result. Or, because tomato plants are pretty harmless (like bifida infantis, the baby bacteria we start off with if we're breastfed) imagine dropping a million blackberry bushes into the same grass land. That's the kind of activity we're engaging in with adding lactobacilli to the gut. In some cases it may really improve the overall conditions, but in no case do we really consistently know the outcome.

Simply not knowing the conditions, would we normally start dropping a million blackberry bushes into a wild grass land or even a rainforest? Not unless we really needed to. But if you could smell the stink of the rotting rainforest, if it was exploding with all sorts of putrid nastiness, you might be well justified in dumping in a few million blackberry bushes in just to see if things don't improve. Because often they will. So when you're in serious trouble, you could do worse than start with even the saddest little commercial lactobacillus probiotic. It might help.

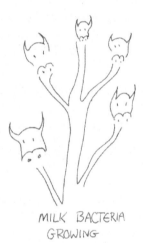

MILK BACTERIA
GROWING

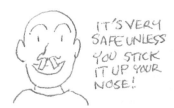

IT'S VERY SAFE UNLESS YOU STICK IT UP YOUR NOSE!

23

TRYING A YEAST

My current favorite starting probiotic species is Saccharomyces boulardii. Unlike the milk bacteria supplement free-for-all, S. boulardii was generated specifically for immune compromised individuals who had issues with antibiotics. As such, it generally outperforms lactobacillus mixes that were originally bred to make yogurt rather than survive our inner rainforests. (Unless the lactobacillus was bred specifically for situations like kidney failure, which is a growing field.)

The origin of S. boulardii was the recognition of the constant yeast infections of AIDS patients. These immune-compromised patients needed multiple doses of antibiotics to stay alive, but suffered horribly from the resulting Candidal yeast infections. (Candida gut infection remains a controversial diagnosis for the "healthy' rest of the population.) As a result, researchers looked for and found S. boulardii, a member of the beer yeast family. S. boulardii lives in the same circumstances as Candida and competes with it for space and food. The result continues to be better outcomes for AIDs patients.

What else can S. boulardii do? It reduced adult antibiotic-induced diarrhea in a Spanish study and has been shown in multiple studies to be helpful with childhood diarrhea. When used with Crohns or Ulcerative Colitis, it improved symptoms in both. In patients with ulcers, S. boulardii helped them get better faster.

Those looking for an easy answer: "let's all take S. boulardii, every day, all the time" are mistaken. In one study, elderly patients did not have their antibiotic-induced diarrhea improved by S. boulardii. A closer look at the study shows that S. boulardii caused diarrhea and made outcomes worse than nothing. One of the biggest issues is that an allergic response to S. cerevisiae, the beer yeast cousin of S. boulardii, can show up in patients with inflamed guts. In that case, it's possible to cross-react to S. boulardii, and your probiotic friend becomes just another cause of diarrhea.

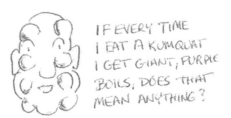

IF EVERY TIME
I EAT A KUMQUAT
I GET GIANT, PURPLE
BOILS, DOES THAT
MEAN ANYTHING?

24

USING SPECIFIC SEED TO COMBAT
INFECTIONS

My favorite yeast, S. boulardii, was created to combat Candida yeast infections. But few other species have been considered as possible treatments for human diseases. The model is still based on more antibiotics, which only modify the internal garden without sterilizing it. Only when antibiotics or other killing treatments are no longer an option do medical doctors consider alternatives. In malaria, which has become resistant to most drugs in some parts of the world, researchers are considering altering the internal gardens of the mosquitoes themselves. If you add a probiotic to the mosquitoes, it interferes with the growth of malaria and solves the problem at the source. Now we just need to get the mosquitoes to eat their probiotics.

BACTERIA PARATROOPERS

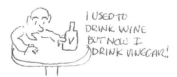

25

TRYING A BLEND

If S. boulardii seems familiar, it's likely that at some point you've been exposed to Kombucha tea, a fascinating process that involves growing your own fermented tea bath. One of the central pieces of this bath is S. boulardii, though there are many other species present. All Kombuchas are not identical, and those considering growing their own should do so with care. Fortunately, commercial blends of Kombucha are also now available in health food stores and supermarkets. Unfortunately, they are widely divergent in the amount and quantity of the species available.

Many other "blends" are available, including most of what we think of as fermented food of any kind. The classic example is yogurt, which is often where most people's knowledge of probiotics begins and ends. A consumer reports analysis found that all yogurts contain a range of living lactobacillus species. It doesn't matter whether you get the store brand or the expensive brand. That's a better bet than a probiotic capsule, which may or may not have enough of what it says it has inside. Consumer Labs found some probiotics capsules contained 16% of what they said they did. Even if you have a good yogurt doesn't mean it will grow in your gut. A study of Bulgarian homemade yogurt found one species of lactobacilli that survived the stomach acid well and grew effectively in the guts of volunteers. But that species isn't anywhere on a commercial yogurt blend label.

It's worth noting that a homemade yogurt blend is an entirely different mix that something from a commercial shop. The same goes for anything fermented, including sauerkraut, which is commonly the only other fermented food familiar to a standard American diet. Unfortunately many commercial sauerkrauts have "flavor added" rather than containing the original fermenting bacteria. An original fermented sauerkraut may also contain lactobacillus species, but ones that may be more resistant to stomach acid.

As we move farther away from a standard American diet, we come across fermented foods like Chinese sauerkraut. There are more exotic names: Kimchi, Gundruk, and Sinki (an article on fermentation list twenty-nine well-known products and briefly describes their preparation). Kimchi or Kim Chee is a Korean sauerkraut using Nappa cabbage and cayenne and is popular enough to be found in standard grocery stores. Gundruk is a Nepalese sauerkraut that is traditionally buried in the earth and contains less salt. Sinki is similar, but made from the roots of radishes. Just about any vegetable seems to used somewhere as a base for fermentation. All of these "sauerkrauts" use lactic acid species in the family lactobacillus but the species vary enormously throughout the world. While we have little research on many species, Chinese sauerkraut contains lactobacillus species that may consume fats and possibly lower overall cholesterol. So if you are looking for a different lactic-acid based batch of "seeds," any Asian market would be good starting place. All of the species have survived in an acidic environment, making them more likely to survive the stomach acid and take root in the gut. But the dried form of many finished products may have killed off bacterial colonies, as would anything covered in chemical preservatives.

Moving even farther afield, we have miso soup, prepared with a stock and soybeans fermented with Aspergillus oryzae (except red miso, produced by M. Purpureus, known in the U.S. as red rice yeast extract). The fungus A. oryzae is used to ferment soy sauce, rice vinegars, and sake (Japanese wine). A Japanese study of miso soup's effects found no change in their subjects internal gardens, but in Japan A. oryzae is so common it is found in nasal passages so it is likely their subjects were already exposed. Pigs fed a mix of probiotics including the Bulgarian yogurt bacteria and A. oryzae showed improvement in overall gut species though none of the original probiotics remained (the same effect we noted in adding S. boulardii to antibiotics). Another Japanese fungi, Rhizopus oryzae, is used making tempeh, a nutty-tasting soybean cake. While extremely safe, R. oryzae was the cause of a single reported case of sinusitis.

Lest we think that only the Japanese consume fungus, let's return to our European fascination with aged, molded proteins that we consume with grapes and fine wine: cheese. Cheese is officially produced using lactobacillus species, but soft cheeses like Camembert also use mold to soften the cheese after it's been hardened. In reality, creating something that sits around for months like a cheese means that most ordinary cheeses contain mold or fungi. In a study of fungi in cheeses, the yeast Debaryomyces hansenii was found in the majority of commercial cheeses. Eighteen other fungi were found, and Penicillium roqueforti mold was found in many cheeses, not just Roquefort cheese. D. hansenii is a more robust yeast than S. cerevisiae because it can tolerate more salt, and subspecies have been found in arctic glaciers. In small-scale, traditionally-made cheeses, D. hansenii is only sometimes the dominant yeast, and its addition to Camembert cheeses can reduce the diversity of other species. So even as we become aware of the diversity of fungi and yeasts in cheeses, that diversity is declining with mass commercial production. Still, having a soft cheese is a sure-fire way to add D. hansenii to your gut. D. hansenii is part of the internal garden of the majority of the world's population, and many of the world's fishes. While D. hansenii has caused a few cases of hospital infection, lab reports show that D. hansenii (also known as Candida famata) may be mistaken for its more aggressive cousin, Candida albicans, well known to women for causing yeast infections the world over. What else comes with the D. hansenii in your cheese? No one knows for sure, and a French study of cheeses came back with over a hundred different bacteria, including several previously unknown (in comparison, U.S. cheeses are very uniform - too much sanitation).

No discussion of blends would be complete without a mention of apple cider vinegar. Not the sterilized, empty acidic vinegars that fail to do anything other than act as a flavoring and cleaning agent. These are the vinegars with the mother swirling down at the bottom, bacteria so numerous and dense they form clouds of material visible to the naked eye. While apple cider vinegar has been studied for cholesterol lowering effects, relatively few human studies have been done on either vinegar or the acetobacter, the bacteria that forms the vinegar. The presumption is that, like soft cheeses, apple cider vinegar has undergone two fermentations. The first fermentation by either bacteria or yeast produced alcohol (hard cider). The second fermentation turns that alcohol into vinegar (which is avoided in wines by blocking air and adding sulfites). So apple cider vinegar contains more than one organism and acts as a blend.

26

HUMAN COMPOST TEA?

When organic gardeners talk about miracle products, they get into a fermented frenzy over a thing they call "compost tea." While different gardeners use different blends, Teaming with Microbes authors Jeff Lowenfels and Wayne Lewis recommend a compost mix that has been aerated by a fish tank blower to maintain a good blend of bacteria that prefer oxygen.

Aeration may work well in the soil, but it's more questionable in the body. Arguably, we've been trying to do the job of increasing diversity using only a couple of air-breathing species, and most of those prefer milk as a food source. It's time to start branching out into the anaerobic species to repopulate the "middle layer" of our internal garden.

As Lowenfels and Lewis point out in their book, anaerobic fermentation does not favor bacteria, it favors fungi. And because we're in the stone ages about gut fungi, we have no real idea what is in there and how to support it. While manufacturers may change in the future, currently we have one yeast (S. boulardii) and no fungi on the supplement market being marketed in capsule form as probiotics.

The closest thing we have to human compost tea is kombucha tea. Even the name of this tea varies greatly, as do the individual ingredients of the bacteria and yeast that form the "mushroom," a mat of bacteria and yeast that forms on the top of the tea like a fungus. (The official mushroom name is delightfully Seussian sounding: zooglea.) While individual reports claim it solves everything, research is sparse and covers the chemical ingredients of the tea rather than treating it like a bacterial/yeast soupy compost tea. The Mayo clinic warns that poor brewing practices can lead to problems, but rat studies show no toxicity from kombucha at very high quantities.

Are all kombucha comparable? Probably not. Michael Roissin analyzed over a thousand samples of kombucha and concluded that "(b)ecause each ferment is unique, we do not want to give the impression that your ferment is going to provide the constituents we have isolated..." so no two kombuchas are the same. Mr. Roissin also warns that conditions of fermentation affect the mix profoundly: "we have noted the effects of various types of stress on the colony. The bacteria and yeasts in a ferment appear to "remember" what environmental stresses have been imposed on them." His book, Analysis of Kombucha Ferments, amounts to a kombucha brewery science manual (complete with lots of chemistry and lab results).

Can Kombucha be improved on? Some researchers argue for the addition of lactobacillus species to improve its health effects but focused on the increased antibiotic function of lactobacillus on other species. Other researchers are using different bases, recognizing that the core ingredients of Kombucha (black tea and sugar) are not the only fermentable compounds. Using whey protein gave a non-carbonated Kombucha-like mixture. Given the historical proliferation of lactic acid bacterial fermentation to seemingly every possible vegetable, it simply makes sense that we need that level of individuality in different kombucha mixes. Fashion designers are even working with the cellulose portion (the zooglea "mushroom") and thinking about how we could use that to make clothing. (Hint: the high vinegar content of the "cloth making" kombucha doesn't make for tasty drinking.)

Other human "compost teas" exist, including Chinese ripe Pu-erh tea, which would provide an interesting mix of fungi. But because the fermentation process is somewhat uncontrolled, there have been complaints of poor quality ripe Pu-erh that has been contaminated by possible disease-causing species. Analysis has shown no contamination, and the species involved are almost entirely fungal instead of the yeast/bacteria blend of kombucha. As Lowenfels notes, some plants like bacteria, others prefer fungus. You will need to experiment to find out which your internal garden prefers.

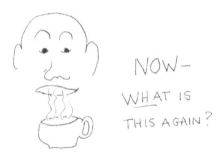

27

STARTING SMALLER:
LESS GROSS COMPOST TEAS

Some farming types have already scampered off to brew their own teas, but many non-farmers react to a human compost tea the same way they would react to "grow your own poop in a jar." It's pretty gross if you aren't used to shoveling manure.

Do not despair. The French have your back. Rather than compost tea, you'll be sampling fine French cheeses (or selected Danish, English, or Irish blends). This only applies if you are in

North America. If you're reading from Europe, then you'll be sampling fine, small-scale organic American cheeses. I use the term organic loosely, as most American goat cheeses or specialty cheeses will do. We're just not interested in mass-produced cheeses unless they happen to be a soft cheese (camembert, etc.) from another continent. Most mass-produced cheeses use the same culture, and are likely already in your system. The soft cheeses have at least the bacteria and a secondary mold, giving you a minimum blend. A smaller, boutique cheese will have a unique signature of micro-and myco-biome to give it the unique taste and you the unique exposures.

Consuming one to two ounces of fine foreign cheese with your meals is hardly a difficult prescription. Just be sure to watch the effect and record it and the brand of cheese for the future.

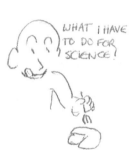

28

GETTING PERSONAL:

CREATING AN INTERNAL GARDENING PLAN

Since every garden is unique, it is impossible to make an absolutely true statement other than: wide variations will exist. Maybe, like snowflakes, you can eventually find an identical match for your microbiome in all the people in the world (who is also likely your soulmate). But for the most part, you will need to engage in surveillance. It's time to to do an internal garden stake-out.

Adding More

Oh, I meant steak-out (groan). No seriously, go out and have a steak. Record your reactions that day and the next to a standard American meal. If you don't react, great. If you find yourself groggy like too many shots of Tequila in your college years, then break down what you ate into individual items and try them individually. Maybe it wasn't the steak, it was that nasty bean dip or the potato salad. (Hint: for microbiologists, it's always the potato salad. Watch them skirt it like a landmine at picnics, their minds full of bacteria chewing on the egg in the sun-warmed salad and multiplying.)

If the steak-out didn't bother you, try out a Thai-out. Usually Thai food is a love/hate relationship, because it's so close to the health food we think we should be eating. Either you feel gypped and vaguely uneasy, or you love that it still tastes pretty good.

How about a Chinese-out, a Mex-out, or a German-out? You get the idea. We're introducing meals, seeing how you react to different foods while quietly expanding the fertilizers you take in. An internal garden that has only been exposed to a few foods doesn't know what it's missing and can't ask for what it really wants. One of my favorite dishes sounds like a children's nonsense nursery rhyme: Ok Dol Bi Bim Bap. But I only found out I loved it by trying the strangest thing on the menu. And it really was, a traditionally Korean dish being served in a Thai restaurant. True, that sense of exploration also led me to eating cow's hoof soup in an Ethiopian restaurant (soaked, gelatinous hoof is still hoof) but I lived to talk about it. Besides, I was just so thrilled to be eating anything Ethiopian, I didn't mind (who knew they had food, much less a distinctive ethnic cousine?).

Once you've figured out what makes you happier, incorporate those new foods into your life. We know that diversity is the best route to a happy bowel, and having more diverse fertilizers can only help. Ideally, your craving for that amazing Indian pancake or that German sausage will be consistent with what's best for your body.

Going Traditional

As a genetic mutt, I can't claim one ancestral genetic line. But if you can trace a fair portion of your heritage to one area or region, then it is worthwhile to explore eating traditional foods prepared in the original style. For example, a portion of my heritage is French, so I would think eating more along the lines of a Frenchman might be beneficial. It might not, but the attempt might lead to a few new foods I enjoy.

Doing Less

For some people, even the idea of going out to a new restaurant is unthinkable. Any variation from three or four meals at home or at their favorite "American food" restaurant just doesn't sit right with them. For those, we have the elimination diet (see Appendix

A) where they single out individual foods to avoid to see if it makes them feel better. Typically, adding a food back into the diet in large quantities will either trigger a response or it won't. It's less fun than adding more foods, but can give you a better sense of what does and doesn't bother you.

Bringing In A Probiotic

Rather than immediately starting with a capsule, it may be best to start with an individual probiotic.

With the discussion of compost tea, many of you may want to start with Kombucha, but be very cautious about your supplier if you are "inheriting" another person's homegrown mixture. The commercial blends of Kombucha cause me to ferment, but I have patients who have completely resolved years of issues by drinking the commercial blends regularly. As I noted in our discussion of Kombucha, different blends lead to different mixes. I'm sure there's a "compost tea" out there for me, I just haven't found it and I may have to make my own.

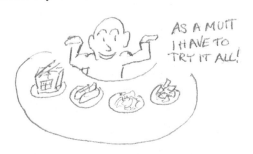

29

MAKING PERSONAL CHOICES
AND UNDERSTANDING YOUR OWN
COMPLEXITY

Given the French portion of my background, I was intrigued by the soft cheese possibility. My experience with cheeses made in the U.S. I've documented over several years in my weight studies. It's constipating and unfortunate. But I also have a history of working at a cheese farm, where they made goat cheeses. So perhaps I was sensitized to the cultures they used to make cheeses in the U.S.?

The experiment of eating non-U.S. cheeses is continuing. While not constipating, my concern is that there are still possibly inflammatory results from adding cheese to my diet. It's too early to tell whether the cheeses are beneficial or just yummy. But I'll forage on in my fromage experiment for the sake of the good of humanity! Since smaller portions don't seem to make any large difference, I'll need to work up my courage to increasing the dosage and seeing if they are still on the "no-fly" list of foods. Rather than considering me squeamish, realize that the common Roquefort cheese growing mold, Penicillium roqueforti, is the same mold that contaminates grain samples and may cause neurotoxicity in animals. I just need to hope my particular cheese strain is low in those compounds, as the levels vary widely and one of the compounds in the cheese might injure dogs. Officially, my exposure is low enough in commercial cheeses to not be concerned. I might even get some antibiotic action from my cheese.

In an update of the paragraph above, I did binge on soft French cheeses in Quebec (ah, the trials I must endure!) and did wonderfully until I ran into a crepe full of American Swiss. The reaction was immediate and troubling. I felt a tingle in my upper throat, and almost had difficulty breathing for a few minutes. Not something I would want to repeat. In the future, I will ask the origin of my cheeses.

My final update is less than enthusiastic. While I can eat French cheeses, over time daily cheese consumption constipates. I can still indulge occasionally, but I can't make even French cheese a daily staple.

We all need to have that level of awareness to truly remain healthy in modern society. Gone are the days of a semi-tribal community where the whole group takes care of each other. Even family doctors have become largely nomadic, and may transfer patients without a second thought as to continuity. The only person who can truly know your body is you, but that knowledge only arises after carefully watching how you react over time. While changes occur in the body over time, remember that individuals can return to balance despite antibiotics, illness, or other assaults on the internal garden.

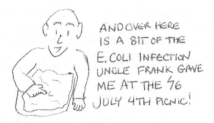

AND OVER HERE IS A BIT OF THE E. COLI INFECTION UNCLE FRANK GAVE ME AT THE '76 JULY 4TH PICNIC!

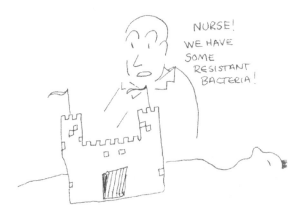

30

DEALING WITH GARDEN PESTS

The reality is that, knowing everything we do about the individualized complexity of our bodies, we can still recognize a massive overgrowth of a single species. In those situations, we may need to do more than simply change fertilizer (although the dietary modification remains the key to lifelong results).

When infected, do seek standard care. Our system of medicine evolved around sudden illness and its resolution. I would much rather see a patient for the side effects of modern medicine than see them continuing to try and unsuccessfully home-treat an out-of-control issue. To paraphrase an old joke, sometimes God sends a miracle, and sometimes just a boat. Take the boat, get better, and deal with the consequences afterward. There are a couple of more and more common situations that may not respond to standard therapies that I'll talk about briefly here.

Candida

Generally, using S. boulardii either orally or topically (capsules dissolved in warm water) will compete with candida directly. The symptoms should clear quickly. If not, you have my permission to bring out the flamethrower (antifungal). Just be sure to also take additional thiamine to offset the possible side effects. Follow-up with an alkaline supporting diet (fruits and vegetables) to get your body back into balance.

MRSA

While Methicillin-resistant Staphylococcus aureus (MRSA) is an ever-expanding problem for anyone depending on antibiotics, it is less intractable if you look at other options. Adding S. boulardii to Vancomycin treatment (for hospitalized patients) may be helpful. But we are beginning to see VRSA, Vancomycin resistant MRSA, which is largely untreatable and all that is left is to watch and wait to see if the patient can overcome the infection on his or her own. It is virtually unknown in other parts of the world, but accounts for up to 2% of cases in parts of the U.S. As it has with MRSA, we expect that percentage to rise over time.

Even as modern medicine can see the grim possibility of untreatable infections mounting, alternatives remain largely unexplored. In an effort to become "more scientific" researchers have forgotten that most existing antibiotics were discovered from plant sources through a process called "bioprospecting." The few synthetic compounds don't have the same reach and use as those created by natural sources. Allicin, for example, can effectively block MRSA, but remains unused in hospitals despite its widespread use everywhere else. (Allicin is the active compound in garlic and onions.) For topical use, dermatologists are returning to gentian violet after other drugs fail. To paraphrase Robert Frost, perhaps our ending the pursuit of more perfect drugs will be the beginning of our return to where we started. We will no longer ignore our roots (and flowers), but truly know them and appreciate them for the first time.

If we acknowledge that new pests will continue to create problems, and recognize that the best solutions we have will likely be old ones, then the rise of something like VRSA becomes a greater call for individualized compost tea and a greater focus on your own internal garden.

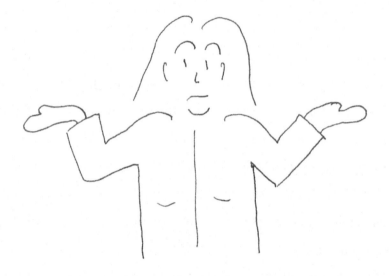

31

WHERE DO I GO FROM HERE?

If your mind is reeling with too much information, don't be concerned about remembering it all. The microbiome is a vast new frontier, and in the next few years we may learn things that completely contradict much of what we think we know about medicine as a whole.

It's really worthwhile to take stock of your personal situation before changing anything in your microbiome. If your bowels are happy, content, peaceful, regularly moving with "banana" poops that float, please don't embark on a massive overhaul. The system is fine, you don't need to do anything.

But let's say you've got a bit of an issue. Gaseous clouds that periodically pollute your bathroom and drop pigeons outside. Nothing terrible, just not pleasant. Then start with an exploration of what might work better for you. Chapter 28 is the place to start, changing your daily "fertilizer" around before you add in any new probiotics. It's always best to add "for the rest of your life" to any supplement or probiotic you're considering taking. Many of us might try an expensive pill for a month, but wouldn't invest our lifesavings in maintaining a supply for twenty more years. But you will need to eat twenty years from now. Exploring now may save you and others around you in twenty years when you can't move fast enough to escape your own gas clouds.

If your problem is more major, then it's time to get someone else involved. Have a conversation with a health provider you trust. Make sure that your issue isn't something worse than bowel imbalance.

Once you've been cleared of anything major, start with Chapter 28. If you want to do a standard elimination diet, I've included one as Appendix A. Figure out how far food can take you and then expand into the range of probiotics. Plan to try several before deciding on one. If you are more hands-on, work with the probiotic foods. Eventually, you may need to get or make your own human compost tea. Only work within your comfort zone, and get the help you need to move forward.

Finally, applaud yourself! You now know more than almost everyone you know, PhD and doctor alike, about the human microbiome. Spread the word, and help heal the planet.

Happy gardening!

APPENDIX A

ANTI-INFLAMMATORY DIET

The following is lifted, with minor variations, from Dr. Dick Thom, an instructor at NCNM. While he told us it was fine to take and make changes to, the credit belongs with him.

Eat only the following organically grown foods for 21 days
Steamed vegetables:
Eat a variety of any and all vegetables that you tolerate. Avoid tomatoes, potatoes, eggplant and bell peppers. Yams, sweet

potatoes, and squash are allowed. The primary reason for using steamed vegetables is that steaming improves the utilization or the availability of the food substances and it reduces the irritating residue in the gut, allowing it to restore itself.

Nuts

Any nut that you can tolerate except peanuts (actually a legume).

Legumes

Eat a variety of any legumes you are able to tolerate: split peas, lentils, kidney beans, pinto beans, soybeans, mung beans, garbanzo beans, aduki & azuki beans.

Grains

Eat one to two cups of cooked grains per day of those you tolerate. Allowed grains are: millet, basmati or brown rice, quinoa, barley, buckwheat, oatmeal, and amaranth. Other grain foods that may be eaten are rice crisps and wasa crackers. In general, plan meals so that bread is not required (rice and beans instead of tacos, celery and nut butter or a chicken salad instead of a sandwich).

Fish

Deep sea fish is preferred (salmon, halibut, cod, sardines, tuna, mackerel - no shellfish or swordfish). The fish should be poached, baked, steamed, or broiled.

Chicken/Turkey

Eat only white meat and do not eat the skin. The chicken should be baked, broiled, or steamed. Free-range or organic chicken is preferable.

Fruit

Eat 1 or 2 pieces of practically any fruit except citrus. Apples, pears, bananas, U.S. grapes, peaches, apricots, mangos, papayas are all acceptable. If possible, bake the fruit for easier digestion.

Sweeteners

Very small amounts of maple syrup, rice syrup, barley syrup and honey may be used.

Absolutely no sugar, Nutrasweet, or any other sweetener is allowed. Often sugar cravings can be avoided by eating protein with each meal.

Butter/Oils

For butter, mix together 1 pound of butter and 1 cup of extra virgin olive oil (from a new dark jar). Whip at room temperature and store in the refrigerator. Provides the benefits and taste of butter and essential fatty acids. Use extra virgin olive oil for all other situations requiring oil.

Herbal teas and good water to drink

Drink 8 to 10 glasses of clean water every day. Drink 2 to 4 cups of herbal tea, sipped slowly in the evening.

For the time-being, avoid the following foods:

Dairy products (milk, cheese, yogurt, kefir). Eggs. Fried foods. Processed foods. Wheat products (breads, muffins, doughnuts, etc.). Corn products (chips, tacos, enchiladas). All caffeinated products. If necessary, wean down with green tea. Alcohol of all kinds. Potatoes, tomatoes, eggplant, green and red bell peppers. Citrus (grapefruit, oranges, lime, lemon). Peanuts and peanut butter (substitute almond butter if necessary). Meat - red meat and especially pork and pork products. Sugar, Nutrasweet, and all sweeteners (except maple syrup and honey)

Week Menu

The biggest change in many diets is in breakfast. Experiment with having "dinner" in the morning, either prepared the night before or made fresh.

B-Oatmeal (add sunflower or flax, dried fruit), L-chicken salad, fruit, D-rice and beans.

B-Protein smoothie (banana, protein powder, other fruit), L-leftover rice and beans, D-baked salmon and salad.

B-alternative grain cereal with soy milk, Snack-almonds, L-california rolls/sushi, D-bean soup.

B-rice and lentils, L-buckwheat soba, D-Indian curry over rice with steamed vegetables.

B-almond butter on rice toast, L- soy cheese on rice crackers, D-chicken with sweet potatoes.

B-spaghetti squash with raisins, maple syrup, and cinnamon. L-split pea soup D-Stir fry.

B-barley soup L-chicken with steamed vegetables D-Thai take out with baked apples (cinnamon and maple syrup) for dessert.

A change in diet means a opening a whole new world. In reexamining our food, we reexamine our past and our present. Unconscious habits, learned early in childhood, become conscious. An unexamined plate is not worth eating.

ABOUT THE AUTHOR

Dr. Christopher Maloney works very hard to change everything he understands about the world based on what new information is uncovered. He is thrilled by the microbiome and is still working hard to understand the ramifications for health and disease.

Made in the USA
Columbia, SC
28 July 2023

20975170R00065